M C CORTES

10 Day Detox Plan To A Healthier Body

How Detoxing Helped Me Alleviate Inflammation and Shed Excess Weight

*Dedicate this first book to my Husband, who always encourages me
to follow my dreams.
I also want to thank my Lord and Saviour Jesus Christ, who has
blessed me with the best husband and for giving me the strength to
not give up.
To my wonderful children Abraham, Alejandra, and Nicole.
To my wonderful friends who are a strong support and great
cheerleaders.*

Contents

1

Introduction

Congratulations! You've made a fantastic decision to prioritize your health and embark on a journey towards a better you. Whether you're grappling with inflammation, pain, weight challenges, or a combination of these, know that you're not alone. By picking up this guide, you've taken the crucial first step, and you're exactly where you need to be.

I'm thrilled to share with you this 10-Day Detox Plan, crafted to assist individuals, like yourself, who are grappling with inflammation-related issues. Inflammation can stem from various sources, including:

- Excessive medication
- Menopause
- Poor dietary habits
- Toxin exposure (an unfortunate reality in today's world)
- Being overweight
- Dealing with conditions like diabetes.

My motivation for sharing this plan is deeply personal. Having traversed my healing journey, I understand the significance of detoxifying the body to achieve cellular-level cleanliness and balance, from rejuvenating the liver to supporting the lymphatic system.

Toxins lurk everywhere, from the environment to the food we consume, even in our everyday cleaning products and personal care items. Often unknowingly, we subject ourselves to these toxins day in and day out, resulting in inflammation and a myriad of other health issues.

Through my own experiences, I've encountered a battlefield within the medical community. On one side, there are doctors striving to empower patients towards wellness through lifestyle changes like healthy eating and exercise, often facing criticism. On the other side, some physicians tend to lean heavily on prescriptions, viewing diseases as incurable and only manageable through medication, neglecting the potential of holistic approaches.

Interestingly, while some doctors dissuade patients from exploring alternative medicine practitioners such as acupuncturists, chiropractors, or functional medicine doctors, I encourage you to keep an open mind. What do they fear? Perhaps the possibility of patients achieving true wellness and merely needing annual check-ups. But isn't that a goal worth pursuing?

If you're tired of merely managing symptoms with maintenance medication and yearn to rid yourself of the underlying issues, seeking alternative medical guidance might be a path worth considering. *I'm not advocating for any specific approach*; I'm sharing insights gleaned from my journey.

While scientific literature on detoxing may be sparse, and opinions may vary, I can offer you my firsthand experience and insights into various detox methods. *Ultimately*, the choice rests with you—to take charge of your health and do what feels right for your well-being.

The plan I'm about to unveil is one that I've personally completed and found immensely beneficial. In the chapters ahead, I'll delve into my reasons for embarking on this detox journey.

My goal is simple: to see you succeed, feel vibrant, and maintain a positive outlook as you strive towards a healthier version of yourself.

Always remember, "You were fearfully and wonderfully made." So, without further ado, let's embark on this transformative journey together.

A Quick Disclaimer Notice:

This book offers health, wellness, and nutritional information and is designed for educational purposes only. You should not rely on this information as a substitute for, nor does it replace, professional medical advice, diagnosis, or treatment. If you have any concerns or questions about your health, you should always consult with a physician or other healthcare professional. Do not disregard, avoid, or delay obtaining medical or health-related advice from your healthcare professional because of something you may read in this book. Consult with your physician before beginning any exercise program, or making any significant changes to your diet, such as by using any supplement, nutrition plan, or meal replacement product. It is your responsibility to ensure that you are following all safety instructions and listening to your body while doing this detox plan.

2

Why Detox - My Story

There is an overwhelming abundance of information available on the internet regarding detox methods. Amidst this sea of opinions and data, sifting through to find reliable, factual information can be a daunting task. Yet, it was a journey I undertook to reach the place where I stand today.

Some may debate the efficacy and safety of detoxification, with differing perspectives on how and when it should be done. However, from my personal experience, I can attest to its transformative power. It played a pivotal role in my journey back to wellness, particularly in alleviating the chronic inflammation and challenges brought on by menopause. While some may attribute my symptoms solely to menopause, I discovered that the root cause lay deeper. It wasn't just menopause; it was the cumulative effect of years of poor dietary choices and toxin exposure that manifested once my estrogen levels began to decline.

What I share with you is my journal, chronicling my experience with a 10-Day Detox Plan. This plan catalyzed my transition to a healthier lifestyle, enabling me to rid my body of the chronic inflammation that had plagued me for so long.

Allow me to offer a glimpse into my life. I'm a mother of three wonderful home-schooled children and married to an extraordinary man who happens to be a Chiropractor and health enthusiast. Together, we've crafted a life filled with blessings, from nurturing our children to pursuing outdoor adventures and creating cherished memories. However, as I reached the age of 52, my body began to betray me.

Initially, minor signs developed into a multitude of health hurdles, leaving me feeling utterly perplexed and demoralized. Simple activities like eating became a challenge, with persistent bloating and weight gain despite my efforts to maintain a healthy diet. Frustration reached its peak when I embarked on a 5K training regimen, only to be sidelined by excruciating pain in my heel and subsequent joint discomfort. Determined not to succumb to despair, I delved into research, seeking solutions to cleanse my body at a cellular and glandular level.

Amidst my quest for answers, I stumbled upon research from the National Institutes of Health (NIH), shedding light on the limited studies surrounding detoxification programs. Despite the lack of conclusive evidence, numerous success stories underscored the potential benefits of detoxing.

In my pursuit, I discerned the distinction between acute and chronic inflammation and their profound impact on health. Chronic inflammation, often insidious, can precipitate a host of debilitating conditions, underscoring the urgency of addressing its underlying causes.

Armed with this knowledge, I resolved to embark on a 10-day detox plan, a decision that yielded remarkable results, including the alleviation of inflammation and significant weight loss.

To those who resonate with my journey, feeling worn down by the ceaseless cycle of sickness and fatigue, I offer a beacon of hope. In the chapters ahead, I will unveil the nourishing foods that propelled my detox journey forward. Remember, resilience remains paramount—despite the hurdles, you are worthy of reclaiming vitality and well-being.

Stay steadfast and determined; your health is a precious gift deserving of diligent stewardship.

3

Planning Ahead & Consistency is Key

Successful individuals across various domains share common traits and practices that contribute to their achievements:

- **Mental Fortitude**: They eliminate all negative reasons that may hold them back.
- **Consistency**: They persistently work towards their goals without giving up.
- **Focus**: They stay focused on their objectives, often by writing them down and keeping them visible.
- **Preparation**: They prepare ahead of time to avoid temptation and stay on track.

At my husband's suggestion, I started by keeping a journal to document my detox journey. This practice allowed me to monitor my weight and track how I felt throughout the process.

My first step was meal preparation. Knowing that hunger could lead to poor choices, I prepped my meals and shakes in advance. Despite living with others who didn't need to detox, I remained steadfast in my commitment to mental fortitude.

I meticulously organized my shakes, dividing ingredients into labeled bags for each day of the 10-day plan. I used 1-gallon zip lock bags to store each daily shake ingredient, you can use whatever is convenient for you. (This is when my OCD kicked in). Additionally, I prepped vegetables for baking or grilling, ensuring I had nutritious options readily available.

Throughout the detox, I primarily consumed shakes, supplemented with vegetables, salads, and plenty of water. I allowed myself green tea or coffee sweetened with monk fruit sugar, steering clear of creamers.

It's important to note that sugar withdrawal symptoms may arise during detox, such as headaches and lethargy. However, these symptoms typically subside within a few days, replaced by increased energy and vitality.

For those on medications, consulting a healthcare professional before embarking on any detox regimen is important. Adjustments to medication may be necessary as the body undergoes healing. Individuals managing conditions like diabetes or high blood pressure must remain vigilant, monitoring their insulin and blood pressure levels throughout the detox process.

Each journey towards wellness is unique, and while my experience centered on healing inflammation and weight loss, your motivations may differ. However, the ultimate goal remains the same: achieving optimal health.

I've provided a comprehensive shopping list and shake recipes for days 1-10 to aid in your preparation.

Remember, diligent preparation and consistency are the keys to a successful detox.

4

Detox Plan Instructions

Embarking on your detox adventure? Let's kick things off with a bang - why not start on a weekend? Picture this: the perfect opportunity to ease into the process, making any necessary adjustments with the luxury of time on your side. There might be days when you don't quite feel like yourself but fret not! Beginning on a weekend grants you the freedom to prepare your meals in advance, setting you up for success.

Now, let's dive headfirst into this journey with enthusiasm and determination!

Your detox journey will revolve around delicious shakes, savored 3 to 4 times a day using the recipes provided in this book. But hey, if hunger strikes, don't hesitate to indulge in additional healthy foods.

Want to elevate your shake game? Consider incorporating a scoop of protein powder. Take your pick between Whey Isolate Protein or pea protein, just be mindful of avoiding sweeteners.

And guess what? A world of diverse fruits and veggies awaits you to elevate your daily shake routine - tantalizing recipes coming your way in the upcoming chapter!

But wait, there's more! You're not confined to shakes alone. You can savor the taste of an egg as your protein, anytime, anywhere. And as for veggies, the options are limitless - raw or cooked, grilled, baked, or steamed. Whip up a mixed green salad with cucumbers, green onions, and celery, drizzle it with vinegar and olive oil, and maybe even throw in some grapes for a burst of flavor.

Hydration is key, folks! Aim for at least 8 glasses of water daily, and that's 8 0z glass, alongside your shakes. Need a caffeine fix? Coffee or tea with Monk Fruit or Stevia is allowed, but remember, nothing beats the hydrating power of good ol' H2O.

Now, about those sweeteners. While Monk Fruit or Stevia are included in some recipes, going without them might be the best option. And don't forget your vitamins and supplements - they're your trusty sidekicks on this journey to wellness.

Feeling the need to chew? Solid veggies, especially greens, are here to save the day. And here's a pro tip: prep is key! Chop and freeze everything in advance, separating them by day for ultimate convenience. But remember, hold off on adding protein powder, water, and sweeteners until the day you'll be enjoying your shakes.

One more thing - if you're hitting the gym during your detox, consider upping your protein intake with options like Salmon or Halibut, grilled or baked, to fuel those workout sessions.

And now, a word on what's off-limits during your detox: no alcohol, no dairy products, no meat, no processed foods, and no sweets. Stick to using water in your shakes for maximum detoxifying power.

So, are you ready to embark on this exhilarating detox journey? Get set, go!

<h1 style="text-align:center">5</h1>

Shopping List - Key Ingredients

The list items below are what you will need for your 10-day detox.

Vegetables

- 2 bags of Spinach
- 1 bag of Kale
- 1 cucumber
- Romaine Lettuce
- Zucchini *
- Yellow Squash *
- Arugula
- Broccoli *
- Celery
- Ginger root
- Turmeric root or powder
- Green onions or scallions *
- Lemon Grass

Fruits

- Banana (Fresh or Frozen)
- Mango (Frozen)
- Papaya (Frozen
- Pineapple (Frozen)
- Strawberries (Frozen)
- 5 Green Apple
- Blueberries (Frozen)
- Lemon
- Raspberries (Frozen)
- Lime
- Pear
- Green Seedless Grapes

Other Ingredients

- Chia Seed
- Flax Seed
- Monk fruit Sugar or Stevia
- Protein Powder Isolate Whey or Pea (whichever is your preference)
- Spirulina (this is optional, you can add it to any of the shakes)

** Purchase these items based on how often you plan to eat them during the 10-day detox. You will cut the vegetables and save them uncooked in the refrigerator. I ate them 3 times a week, so I prepared 3 bowls and stored them in the fridge. I seasoned the one serving I was to cook that day, however, you can season them in advance.*

6

Shake Recipes

Shake Day 1

3 handfuls spinach
1 green apple, cored
1 cup of frozen diced mangos (easy on the blender)
1 cup of frozen strawberries
1 cup of frozen green seedless grapes
2 tablespoons of flaxseed
2 cups of water
Protein Powder
1 Pack or teaspoon Monk Fruit or Stevia (optional)

Shake Day 2

3 handfuls of Spinach or Kale (or you can combine them)
1 banana sliced (frozen is ok) I found them frozen in Walmart
1 cup of frozen blueberries, strawberries or raspberries.
2 tablespoon of Chia Seeds
2 cups of Water
Protein Powder (optional)
1 pack or 1 teaspoon of Monk Fruit or Stevia (Optional)

Shake Day 3

3 handfuls spinach
2 cups of frozen pineapple (I found these in Walmart as well and they're
chopped) so convenient.
1 frozen banana
½ of lime juice
2 tablespoon of Chia Seed
2 cups of water
Protein Powder
1 Packet or teaspoon of Monk Fruit or Stevia (Optional)

This one I liked the most, I called it Caribbean Splash, I still drink this one,
however, after the detox I replaced the water with coconut water.

Shake Day 4
3 handful of Kale
1 Green apple cored
1 peeled orange separated in segments
½ of a peeled lemon
1 tablespoon of ginger grated or minced
Protein Powder
2 cups of water
1 pack or teaspoon of Stevia or Monk Fruit (Optional)

Shake Day 5
3 Handful of Spinach
1 Cup of Frozen Strawberries
½ cup of Frozen Blackberries
½ cup of Frozen Raspberries
2 tablespoon of Flaxseed
Protein Powder
2 Cups of Water
1 packet or teaspoon of Monk fruit or Stevia (Optional)

Shake Day 6
3 Handfuls of Kale or Spinach
1 Cups of Frozen Cherries
1 Cup of Frozen Pineapple
2 tablespoons of Flaxseed
Protein Powder
2 Cups of Water
1 packet or teaspoon of Monk fruit or Stevia (Optional)

Shake Day 7
1 Handfuls of each mix of Arugula, Spinach and Kale
1 green apple cored
1 cucumber peeled
1 tablespoon of minced or grated ginger
¼ cup of Lemon grass
Juice of a Whole Lime
Juice of a Whole Lemon
1 cup of water
1 packet or teaspoon of Monk Fruit or Stevia (Optional)

Shake Day 8
3 Handfuls of Spinach
1 cup of Frozen Papaya
1 cup of Frozen Pineapple
1 Frozen Banana
Protein Powder
2 cups of water
1 packet or teaspoon of Monk Fruit or Stevia (Optional)

Shake Day 9
3 Handfuls of Kale
1 Frozen Pear
½ cup of Frozen Banana
1 cup of Mango
1 tablespoon of Minced or Grated Ginger
2 Cups of Water
1 packet or teaspoon of Monk Fruit or Stevia (Optional)

Shake Day 10

3 Handfuls of Spinach
1 Green Apple Cored
1 Green Pear
1 Cup of Frozen Grapes
Protein Powder
2 Cups of Water
1 packet or teaspoon of Monk Fruit or Stevia (Optional)

7

Exercising During Detox

There's often a debate about whether exercise is advisable during a detox. Questions arise: Is it safe? Should I hold off? This issue is crucial because a detox diet reduces calorie intake and other vital nutrients necessary for energy levels and muscle development during workouts. Scientific studies shed light on this matter, stating, "Exercise aids in detoxification by supporting liver and kidney health, facilitating the body's natural defense mechanisms. Regular physical activity improves lymph fluid circulation, enhancing toxin and bacteria elimination." So, exercise isn't inherently harmful. However, during detox, with the low-calorie intake, caution is warranted to avoid muscle fatigue or adverse effects. Certain exercises can maintain movement without strain.

Recommendations include:

- yoga
- foam rolling
- walking.

Although cycling and jogging may be enticing for some, others might find them too mild due to their low impact. It's essential to listen to your body's cues. If you opt for these exercises, consider boosting your protein and vegetable consumption to support your energy levels.

Exercise during detox can lead to:

- fatigue
- dehydration,
- nausea,
- stomach discomfort,
- and dizziness

These symptoms align with detoxing, so stay hydrated and attuned to your body, proceeding with caution. I initially experienced dizziness, nausea, and fatigue, so I refrained from working out until around day four.

Just a little side note, I started my detox on a weekend, to give my body more time to rest and adapt to any changes it would go through.

It's essential to clarify—I offer no medical advice, merely sharing my experience and research-based methods to alleviate inflammation. Always consult a doctor before embarking on any dietary or exercise regimen.

Here is what some experts say about exercising during detoxing:

Exercising during detoxing can be a topic of debate among experts, as opinions vary depending on the type of detox program, individual health conditions, and fitness levels. Here are some common perspectives:

1. Supporters of Exercise During Detox:
Some experts advocate for light to moderate exercise during detox programs, suggesting that it can help support the body's natural detoxification processes by increasing circulation, sweating out toxins, and promoting lymphatic drainage. Low-impact exercises such as walking, yoga, and swimming are often recommended as they can be gentle on the body while still providing benefits.

2. Caution Advised:
Other experts advise caution when it comes to exercising during detox, especially for those undergoing more intense detox protocols or experiencing significant detox symptoms. Detoxing can sometimes lead to feelings of fatigue, weakness, or dizziness, and intense exercise may exacerbate these symptoms or put undue stress on the body.

3. Listen to Your Body:
Many experts emphasize the importance of listening to your body and adjusting your exercise routine as needed during detox. If you feel energized and capable, light exercise may be beneficial. However, if you feel weak or unwell, it's essential to

rest and prioritize self-care.

4. Consultation with Healthcare Professionals:

Individuals with pre-existing health conditions or those undergoing specific detox protocols should consult with healthcare professionals or qualified experts before starting or continuing an exercise routine. Healthcare providers can offer personalized advice based on individual health needs and goals.

Ultimately, whether to exercise during detox depends on various factors, including the type of detox program, individual health status, and comfort level with exercise. It's essential to approach detoxing and exercise with mindfulness, paying attention to how your body responds and making adjustments as needed.

8

What to Expect

After delving into endless research, all I yearned for was to reclaim a sense of normalcy in my life. Uncertain if a detox would truly make a difference, I found myself becoming my experimental subject, a guinea pig of sorts.

They say desperate times call for desperate measures, and indeed, desperation drove me to seek solutions, not mere theories or medications that merely masked symptoms. No, I craved to unearth the root cause of my chronic inflammation, to address it at its core.

I stumbled upon countless accounts of individuals who had successfully healed their inflammation through dietary interventions. Thus began my quest to discover the right foods that held the power to heal.

First, I turned to the Keto diet, inspired by stories of people weaning off their diabetic and high blood pressure medications. Yet, despite my hopes, neither Keto nor fasting alleviated the inflammation that plagued me.

Undeterred, I pressed on, exploring various dietary approaches. Deep down, I knew that the key lay within the realm of food. Then, unexpectedly, I stumbled upon studies extolling the virtues of detoxifying the liver and kidneys, emphasizing the pivotal role of greens in combating inflammation within the body.

Was I weary? Exhausted, even? Absolutely. I anticipated the fatigue, the headaches, and the nausea that accompanied the initial stages of detoxification. Yet, as my body gradually acclimated to eating clean and healthy, the symptoms and discomfort dissipated.

In short, based on my laborious research and personal experimentation, I can attest that detoxification, coupled with a strategic selection of nutrient-rich foods aimed at combating inflammation, proved to be the remedy I desperately sought.

The results were nothing short of transformative. Shedding 10 pounds was just the beginning. My energy levels soared, my sleep improved, and my digestive issues vanished. No longer plagued by joint pains or inflammation, I found myself experiencing life with renewed vigor and optimism.

To those who may be reading this, holding on to hopes of reclaiming their health and shedding excess weight, I offer this advice: embark on a 10-day detox journey. The rewards are boundless. And if I can achieve such remarkable results with my own set of challenges, then so can you.

9

Whats Next After The Detox

Our paths diverge here, as I'm still charging through my second phase. Remember when I hinted at not halting after the initial 10-day detox? Well, I'm living proof of that commitment. I've embraced a lifestyle filled with vibrant, nutrient-packed greens, continuing the journey toward optimal health.

Now, let's talk about the veggies and fruits that'll keep your momentum going post-detox. These nutritional powerhouses will infuse your everyday meals with vitality and help sustain your healing journey.

- Apple
- Arugula
- Asparagus
- Avocado
- Basil
- Broccoli
- Cilantro

- Cabbage
- Celery
- Cranberries • Cucumber
- Goji Berries
- Grapefruits
- Kale
- Lemon
- Lemongrass
- Mint Leaf
- Pomegranate
- Pineapple
- Strawberries, Blueberries, and Raspberries (Low in Sugar)
- Wheat-grass

The possibilities are boundless, by incorporating these essentials into your diet, you'll simplify the journey. Picture this: I start my mornings with a rejuvenating cup of coffee sweetened with Monk Fruit, paired with a protein-packed shake infused with Spirulina, Chlorella, and the Ultimate Super-food Fusion supplements, all sourced from ZNatural Foods. Trust me, their range of natural powder supplements is a game-changer—worth exploring.

Now, please keep in mind change is not easy, it's not always a walk in the park, but once you dive in and make nourishing your body a habit, you'll be hooked. The sense of empowerment and accomplishment, that comes with taking charge of your health is unparalleled.

As for my routine, mornings are reserved for my signature shake, sometimes switching it up for an evening treat. Throughout the day, I savor two wholesome meals and indulge in a snack—think nuts like Almonds, Walnuts, or Pecans, or perhaps some energizing Goji Berries. And hydration? Well, I've got that covered, aiming to guzzle down half my weight in water daily. Trust me, it's a winning formula—I'm steadily shedding pounds, staying active, and most importantly, feeling phenomenal, also know that adding sea salt to your water helps keep your cells hydrated.

Now, let's address the inevitable adjustment period. When diving into a new diet, especially one vastly different from your norm, your body might need a little time to adapt. So, give yourself that grace period. If at first things feel a bit rocky, consider gentle aids like Metamucil or Psyllium husk, or perhaps soothing digestive teas to ease the transition. And don't forget the golden rule: hydrate, hydrate, hydrate—with a minimum of 64 ounces of water daily. After all, this journey is all about nourishing your body and thriving every step of the way.

10

Questions & Answers

These are some of the most common questions about the 10-day detox plan.

Q. I am a Vegan/Vegetarian.
The 10-Day Detox is 100% vegetarian-friendly. As for the protein you can substitute
the Whey Protein powder for Pea Protein.

Q. Can I make a substitution?
I shared some substitutions you can make on the greens and fruits.

Q. I Am Having Trouble with Bowel Movements. What Can I Do?
Experiencing constipation can often arise as a temporary side effect during the shift from a diet laden with processed foods to one focused on cleansing and natural foods. Like with

any significant dietary change, especially when transitioning to a vastly different eating regimen, your body requires an adjustment period. In the initial days of this transition, it's important to allow your body the time it needs to adapt before jumping to conclusions about the healthiness of the cleansing process.

If you find yourself feeling particularly uncomfortable during this adjustment phase, there are gentle aids available to help ease the transition. Consider incorporating into your routine, natural laxatives like Metamucil or Psyllium husk (avoiding stimulant laxatives) or digestive teas to facilitate smoother adaptation. Also, maintaining adequate hydration is crucial, so try drinking at least 64 ounces of water daily. It's important to note that this recommendation does not include the fluids consumed as part of your detox regimen, such as detox water, smoothies, or other teas. By giving your body the support it needs during this transitional period, you can go through the adjustment phase more comfortably and effectively.

Q. I Am Having Gas/Am Feeling Bloated. Is This Normal?

During the initial days of detox, you may experience digestive issues like bloating, cramping, and flatulence. The severity of these symptoms depends on your colon's condition and your pre-detox diet.

Q. I Am on Day 3 And I Feel A Bit Lethargic. What Should I Do?

Depending on your pre-detox diet, feeling lethargic or fatigued during the 10-day detox period is normal. The body is trying to adjust to a cleaner and less processed way of eating. These effects are stronger if you are consuming large amounts of sugar and processed foods before your detox.

Q. How Much Water Should I Be Drinking?

Please try drinking a minimum of 8 – 8 oz. glasses of water daily to ensure you are hydrated. If your activity/exercise level and heat exposure are higher, your water intake needs to increase.

Q. Can I Have Coffee?

Yes! You can. Try limiting your coffee intake to only 1-2 cups per day. Make sure it is unsweetened (unless using stevia or monk fruit) and take your coffee black.

11

Appendix

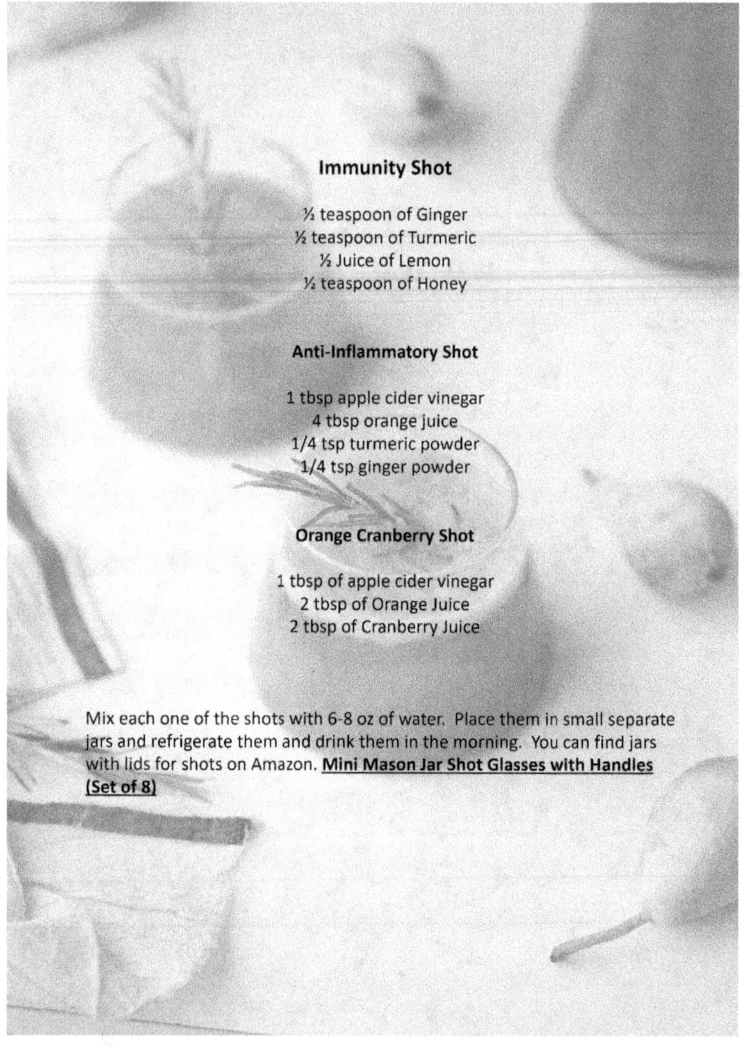

Immunity Shot

½ teaspoon of Ginger
½ teaspoon of Turmeric
½ Juice of Lemon
½ teaspoon of Honey

Anti-Inflammatory Shot

1 tbsp apple cider vinegar
4 tbsp orange juice
1/4 tsp turmeric powder
1/4 tsp ginger powder

Orange Cranberry Shot

1 tbsp of apple cider vinegar
2 tbsp of Orange Juice
2 tbsp of Cranberry Juice

Mix each one of the shots with 6-8 oz of water. Place them in small separate jars and refrigerate them and drink them in the morning. You can find jars with lids for shots on Amazon. **Mini Mason Jar Shot Glasses with Handles (Set of 8)**

12

Resources

Inflammation: What Is It, Causes, Symptoms & Treatment. (n.d.). Cleveland Clinic. https://my.clevelandclinic.org/health/sympto ms/21660-inflammation

"Detoxes" and "Cleanses": What You Need To Know. (n.d.). NCCIH. https://www.nccih.nih.gov/health/detoxes-and-cle anses-what-youneed-to-know

Spritzler, F. (2023, February 16). *Anti-Inflammatory Diet 101: How to Reduce Inflammation Naturally*. Healthline. https://www. healthline.com/nutrition/anti-inflammatory-diet-101#what-it-is

S. (2022, July 2). *The Role of Exercise in Detox: Discover the Truth About Sweating It Out*. Ask the Scientists. https://askthes cientists.com/exerci se-detox/

ZNatural Foods. (2021, October 28). *WHAT ARE THE BEST SUPERFOODS?* https://www.znaturalfoods.com/blogs/articl es/what-are-the-best-s uperfoods.

13

CONCLUSION

In conclusion, it's vital to understand that detoxification can be incredibly beneficial when approached with diligence and adherence to guidelines. Reflecting on my journey, here are the key factors that propelled me toward success:

- Maintain Focus: Keep your eyes on the prize and stay committed to your goals.
- Preparation is Key: Preparing shakes and chopping vegetables in advance sets the stage for seamless adherence to your detox plan.
- Hydration is Vital: Keep yourself hydrated by drinking ample water throughout the day.
- Resist Temptation: Eliminate sources of temptation to stay true to your commitment.
- Prioritize Sleep: Ensure you get sufficient rest, aiming for 7 to 8 hours of quality sleep each night.
- Steer Clear of Daily Weigh-Ins: Avoid obsessing over daily weigh-ins, focusing instead on the bigger picture.
- Visualize Success: Remind yourself of the myriad benefits

awaiting you upon completion of the detox, propelling you towards a healthier, happier lifestyle.

As you embark on your journey, remember to stay centered and unwavering in your dedication to self-care. Preparation and commitment are the cornerstones of success in this endeavor.

I extend my heartfelt wishes for your journey ahead, confident that you too will achieve remarkable results. Stay focused, stay determined, and above all, prioritize your well-being. And if this book has provided value to you in any way, your feedback on Amazon would be greatly appreciated. Thank you for entrusting me with a part of your wellness journey. Here's to your health and vitality!